Ketogenic Diet

The How-To & Not-To

Guide for Beginners:

How to Lose Weight Effectively

By

Orlando Scott

D1532226

Table of Contents

Introduction

Thank you for purchasing the book, *"Ketogenic Diet. The How-To & Not-To Guide For Beginners: How To Lose Weight Effectively"*.

This book contains proven steps and strategies on how to use the low-carb, high-fat Ketogenic Diet as a weight loss method. It is one of the most effective diets for weight loss available today. It's easy to follow and offers many health benefits too. This book offers a guide on what to do and what not to do while following a Ketogenic Diet. It also has guides on how to create diet plans and how to kick-start a workout routine. Keep on reading to know more about all of the above.

Thanks again for purchasing this book, I hope you enjoy it!

Chapter 1
Ketogenic Diet: The Basics

The Ketogenic Diet is an old therapeutic diet developed for the treatment of refractory or difficult-to-control epilepsy in children back in the 1920s. The composition of the diet leads to an elevated level of ketone bodies in the blood which consequently leads to a reduction in the frequency of epileptic seizures. Its revival started in the 1990s and it is now used by many people worldwide.

A Quick Look at Its History

Originally, the Ketogenic Diet was considered part of conventional medicine used to treat epilepsy, but it did not introduce medications in its treatments. Using alternative therapy including fasting, doctors were able to reduce symptoms of pediatric epilepsy. However, due to limitations of fasting therapy, doctors needed a way to improve it. Eventually, the Ketogenic Diet was developed.

Unfortunately, with the discovery of an anti-seizure drug called Phenytoin in 1938, use of the Ketogenic Diet dwindled. Luckily, due to media exposure, including a foundation created by a Hollywood film producer and even a made-for-television film, the diet gained popularity again in the 1990s. In about 1994, a multicenter prospective study kicked off and within the next few years, the results were presented and eventually published by the American Epilepsy Society. Since that period, the Ketogenic Diet has continued to evolve.

The Ketogenic Diet Today

Today, aside from being recognized as an alternative treatment for epileptic seizures, the Ketogenic Diet is known:

- as a low-carbohydrate, high-fat diet

- to offer many health benefits and is also referred to as low-carb high-fat (LCHF) diet, low-carb diet or Keto diet.

The Ketogenic Diet is named after the metabolic state called Ketosis. It is a natural process that the body creates when it experiences low food intake. To induce the process, there is a drastic reduction in carbohydrate intake and a replacement with fats instead. In this state, the body produces Ketones through the liver by breaking down fats and using it for energy. As a result, the body becomes amazingly efficient at burning fat to produce energy and the ketone bodies pass into the brain and become a replacement for glucose as the body's main energy source.

Why Is the Ketogenic Diet Highly Effective?

Eating foods high in carbohydrates causes the body to produce insulin and glucose. Both are important elements that process sugar in the body. Insulin is used to process glucose in the body by distributing it through the bloodstream. Glucose then is also called blood sugar, and since it is already in the blood, the body can easily use it as a primary source of energy. However, because of this, fats in the body are ignored and stored away in places such as the thighs, abdomen, arms and pretty much anywhere.

Eating foods low in carbohydrates meanwhile, causes the body to produce very minimal or even null insulin and glucose. This is no problem because the human body is extremely adaptive and so despite low levels of blood sugar, it still finds a way to produce energy.

With little glucose in the body, it resorts to other sources of energy such as fats. The Ketogenic Diet becomes highly effective in this process because it forces the body to use fats as the primary source of energy by inducing Ketosis.

Different Versions of Ketogenic Diets

Through the years, the Ketogenic Diet has spawned various versions. There is however, a standard and widely-accepted version, which is the subject of this e-book. Here are the various versions of the Ketogenic Diet:

- *The Cyclical Ketogenic Diet (CKD)*

  It is called cyclical because this version involves alternating periods of higher-carb refeeds. For example, there's 2 days of high-carb intake followed by 5 days of the Ketogenic diet.

- *The Targeted Ketogenic Diet (TKD)*

  It is called "targeted" because this version designates workout days as high-carb days. It allows a person to add carbs to their diet during such days.

- *High-Protein Ketogenic Diet*

  This version is a low-carb, high-protein, high-fat diet. The ratio is often 10% carbs, 30% protein and 60% fat.

- *And of course, the Standard Ketogenic Diet (SKD)*

The standard diet is the most recommended version of them all. It is very low in carb intake, moderate in protein, and high in fat. A typical meal in this version contains 5% carbs only, 20% protein, and 75% fats.

CKD and TKD are more advanced methods. They are primarily used by athletes and bodybuilders. However, extensive studies have only been applied to high-protein and standard Ketogenic diets.

Chapter 2
Benefits of the Ketogenic Diet

Ketogenic Diet for Weight Loss

Any version of the Ketogenic Diet is an effective weight loss method. In an initial study, it was found that the Ketogenic diet is a far superior method compared to the much recommended and widely accepted low-fat diet. Numerous studies from Australia, US and the UK have already documented results to confirm this claim. They show that people on this diet lost 2.2 – 3 times more weight compared to those who were on a low-fat, calorie-restricted diet.

Another randomized controlled study indicated that individuals assigned to a very low carbohydrate ketogenic diet are able to achieve greater overall weight loss in the long term than individuals on a low fat diet.

Several factors are believed to be responsible for this key benefit. These factors include:

- *Increased Ketones*

    An increase in ketones indicates that the body is using fat as its source of energy, instead of the more readily available glucose.

- *Increased protein intake*

  An increase in protein intake stimulates hormones that stabilize weight control, enhance metabolism and control appetite.

- *Improved insulin sensitivity*

  The body becomes more sensitive to insulin while undergoing a Keto diet. Improved insulin sensitivity enhances metabolism and fuel utilization.

- *Increased fat burning*

  A rapid increase in fat burning is seen in Keto diet practitioners even when they are resting or performing their regular daily activities.

- *Reduced storage of fat in the body*

  Studies suggest that Keto diets reduce fat storage in the body by cutting down the body's process of turning sugar to fat through lipogenesis.

- *Reduced calories*

  Calories play a key role in weight loss. In a Keto diet, the process of converting protein and fats into energy burns additional daily calories. At the same time, the restriction of carb intake also limits food options which can reduce the intake of additional calories as well.

These factors make the body an efficient fat-burning machine. What makes the Ketogenic diet an even more appealing method for weight loss is that it does not require practitioners to track the food they eat or count their calorie intake. At the same time, due to the increased protein intake, practitioners eat less because the diet makes them feel full quickly. This is supported by the hunger hormones ghrelin and leptin, which undergo positive changes in Keto diets.

Studies also show multiple other benefits that accompany the Ketogenic diet. These include:

- ***Improved energy levels***

Practitioners feel more energized because the body is provided with a more reliable source of energy: fats.

- ***Improved cholesterol levels***

Keto diets lower Triglyceride levels which are associated with arterial buildup.

- ***Improved glucose levels***

  Research shows that long-term decrease in LDL (low-density lipoprotein) cholesterol lowers the risk or altogether eliminates blood sugar-related illnesses.

- ***The lowered risk of acquiring certain diseases***

  Studies show that a Keto diet lowers the risk of getting some diseases. Below is a list of other ailments that a Keto diet can help reduce or eliminate.

Ketogenic Diet for Health

Though the Ketogenic diet was originally developed for therapeutic treatment of pediatric epilepsy, it is now used to benefit many other health conditions including the following:

- ***Heart Diseases***

  A Keto diet lowers the risk of heart diseases because it improves factors such as blood sugar, cholesterol levels, blood pressure and body fat.

- *Acne*

  Recent research has discovered that after 12 weeks of a Keto diet, practitioners have fewer acne lesions. This is due to the reduction in intake of processed foods and sugar, which lowers insulin levels. A Keto diet also reduces skin inflammation.

- *Brain injuries*

  A study revealed that a Keto diet aids in recovery after a brain injury. It also reduces damages caused by concussions.

- *Alzheimer's Disease*

  Keto diets delay the progress of this disease and reduce its symptoms.

- *Cancer*

  Studies are currently ongoing where Keto diet is used to slow the growth of tumors and reduce symptoms of cancer.

- *Polycystic Ovary Syndrome (PCOS)*

Insulin, which plays an important role in the development of PCOS, is highly reduced in a Keto diet, thereby alleviating this syndrome.

Although studies of Keto diets for the benefit of these health conditions are still ongoing, it is clear that in general, it can aid with the treatment of insulin-related, neurological and metabolic diseases.

Ketogenic Diet for Physical Performance and Muscle Gain

Non-practitioners often assume that a Keto diet affects physical performance. They are wrong. A recent study of professional gymnasts, who were on Keto diets, revealed that muscle mass remains the same and endurance is not affected after a few weeks of training. Their bodies successfully achieved Ketosis during this period by limiting glucose storage and using fats instead as the main source of energy.

Another study was done on trained cyclists who were fed with a strict diet of high quality fats, proteins and green vegetables. The results were the same as with the gymnasts. Results revealed that a Keto diet only affects performance if practitioners want an explosive workout. In the case of this explosive workout, to add a little boost to performance, practitioners should add more carbs to their diet 30 minutes before a workout.

Keto diets may limit physical performance at the start, but as the body adapts fully to Ketosis, endurance and strength return to normal. For practitioners looking to gain muscle using a Keto diet, the TKD and CKD versions are more appropriate.

Chapter 3
Ketogenic Diet 101: What to Do in a Ketogenic Diet

Start a Diet Plan

A Ketogenic diet revolves around nutrition plans so in order to start one right, it is important to know which foods are allowed for consumption. In other words, a practical and workable diet plan is the first thing a potential Keto practitioner must develop. Here are the most important things to consider in a Keto diet:

1. Because the subject of this e-book is the Standard Ketogenic Diet, 20-30 grams of daily carbohydrate intake is recommended. The general rule is:

   Low-carb (5%) + moderate protein (25%) + high-fat (70%)

   However, the idea in Keto diets is that the more practitioners limit their carbohydrate intake, the quicker they'll be able to achieve Ketosis. They can take between 15-20 grams of carbohydrates only but to be on the safe side, they should start with the general rule above.

2. Humans basically live on carbohydrate-rich foods. In a Keto diet however, practitioners are required to limit carbohydrate intake. To do this successfully, dieters should source them from dairy, nuts and vegetables only. The best choice is always dark, green, leafy veggies. The perfect meal in a Keto diet would include these veggies, some fat and a little side of protein.

3. The most successful Keto diets are the ones low in carbohydrate and glucose or sugar.

4. Important electrolytes, such as sodium, are flushed out quickly when there is little storage of carbohydrates in the body. This happens because there is less water retention in the body, leading to a mineral and water imbalance. Lots of water or salted chicken, beef, or pork broth or stock is also recommended to replace the lost water and sodium. Diet practitioners should drink the daily recommended intake of water as well. Otherwise, dehydration and low levels of electrolytes can lead to panic attacks, headaches and heart palpitations.

Now, what do practitioners have to eat? These foods should be the base of Keto meals:

Foods Allowed in Keto Diets

- *Organically-grown vegetables for source of carbohydrates*

  Low-carb vegetables

  Green, leafy vegetables

  Onions

  Peppers

  Tomatoes

- *Organically-processed dairy for source of carbohydrates, protein and fat*

  Eggs

  Unprocessed cheese such as mozzarella cheese

  Cream cheese

  Goat cheese

  Cheddar cheese

  Cream and butter

- *Meat for source of protein and fat*

    Poultry meat such as turkey and chicken

    Pork such as bacon, sausage, ham and steak

    Beef

    Fatty fish (with Omega-3) such as mackerel, tuna or salmon.

- *Nuts and seeds for source of protein and fat*

    Chia seeds. They are the rave nowadays and are highly recommended because they are loaded with nutrients.

    Pumpkin seeds

    Flaxseeds

    Walnuts

    Almonds

    Peanuts

- *Healthy oils for source of fat*

    Avocado oil

Coconut oil

Olive oil, but the extra virgin variety is highly recommended

- *Fruits*

Avocado

Apricots

Grapefruit

All kinds of berries – blackberries, blueberries, raspberries and strawberries.

Single ingredient foods or whole foods are the best ones to be included in a Keto diet. Condiments, spices and healthy herbs are also recommended because they are good sources of electrolytes which can be lost due to low-carb intake. A more detailed look at foods to eat for Keto diets will be discussed in Chapter 5.

What about fast food or gourmet dining? Are they allowed?

Tips When Dining Out While on a Keto Diet

One of the most common problems of Keto diet practitioners is the fact that they may be invited to dine out with family or friends, or the fact that they may have to go on a romantic date. Restaurants and fast food joints do not always have Keto-friendly foods. The trick to maintain the diet while eating out is to order meat, fish, poultry or egg-based dishes as the main course. Add some veggies for carbohydrates and order berries with cream or cheese for dessert. For more details, here are some tips on what to eat:

1. Many restaurants offer meat, fish, or poultry-based dishes with some carbohydrate-based food on the side. Order any of the three but replace the carbohydrates with vegetables instead.

2. In fast food chains, hamburgers are acceptable and will not ruin the Keto diet but buns should be removed before eating. It should be noted that some fast food chains offer bun-less burgers and these are just perfect. Again, replace the carbohydrates (usually the fries) with vegetables such as salad instead. Order extra cheese, eggs, bacon, or avocado on the side.

3. Egg-based dishes are also an excellent option and should be ordered if possible.

4. For dessert, possible options are cheese and berries with double cream.

How about supplements? Are they allowed in Keto diets?

Supplements Allowed in Keto Diets

Supplements are not necessary in Keto diets. However, they can be useful and can be a source of added nutrients. The following is a list of a few useful supplements that are beneficial when added to a Keto diet.

- Whey – for added protein

- Exogenous ketones and MCT oil – for raising ketone levels in the body

- Caffeine – for added fat loss and performance effects

- Minerals – for replacement of lost minerals, electrolytes and salt

- Creatine – for practitioners who combine Keto diets with exercise

Weight Loss Principles

These weight loss principles could prove to be useful when embarking on a Keto diet.

- ***Weight Control Principle#1: Accountability***

  While Keto sticks are a powerful tool for evaluating the progress of ketosis, the bathroom weighing scale is a helpful tool in determining if weight loss efforts are producing results. On the other hand, Keto practitioners are advised not to be obsessed about their weight but still monitor it once in a while.

  To start, buy a high-quality scale, so that there's no chance that you'll be making false-readings. Check your weight at the same time regularly for example, every Monday mornings before eating breakfast or every Sunday after dinner. This way, there is a more consistent picture of the progress actually being made.

  Keto diets can be used to lose weight quickly in a short period of time. However, there's no need to rush. There's no chance that a Keto dieter can lose 30 pounds in one week because that weight wasn't gained in one week anyway.

People who lose weight quickly can also gain it back quickly so be patient; don't skip meals but enjoy them. Indulge in a low-carb treat or dessert once in a while; these will not hurt because the most important thing is to keep the goal of weight loss in mind.

After achieving the desired weight, do not stop monitoring the diet's progress. Do not put away that weighing scale. It serves both as a tool for motivation and evaluation. It is not an enemy. It is a friend. It's important to learn to see it this way for maximum benefits.

- ***Weight Control Principle#2: Moderation***

Moderation doesn't mean eating until a person is stuffed. It doesn't mean eating until the stomach hurts. It doesn't mean eating as much as the body wants. It means eating fairly and reasonably. This principle should be religiously adhered to if a diet practitioner wants to achieve lasting results.

- ***Weight Control Principle#3: Anti-Slavery***

Slaves have no control over their lives. In weight loss, slavery means an individual who is a bound to food and has no control over when they eat. Do not be one of them.

A Few Basic Changes for Weight Loss

Rules are often seen to be confining and constricting. In reality, following rules often leads to success. Here are a few rules that offer changes that can be applied by Keto practitioners to help them lose weight.

- ### *Rule#1: Start reading labels*

    Many people do not read food labels usually found at the back of food packaging. This is strange because reading labels is more than helpful. When it comes to weight control, many people are on the wrong path simply due to ignorance. They eat haphazardly without considering the source of their weight gain. It's not really a matter of cutting down on food generally but cutting down on those foods that contribute to unhealthy weight gain. For this reason, one must learn the habit of reading labels.

    Many foods today are touted as low-carb or carb-free foods but looking closely at labels, one can see the truth. While shopping for groceries, read each label and compare. Don't just throw anything on the shopping cart. Wise decisions at the grocery store can lead to wise weight loss decisions as well.

- **_Rule#2: Learn how to substitute_**

Fortunately, there is the option of substituting much-loved unhealthy foods with alternative healthy ones. Unfortunately though, not many people practice substitution or are aware of this technique. Little do people know that learning how to substitute certain foods can drastically reduce carb intake. A person simply has to look for ways to replace high-carb foods. For instance, salad dressings can be substituted with olive oil of balsamic vinegar.

- **_Rule#3: Always include snacks in diet plans_**

An unplanned snack is one of the worst enemies of weight loss. Snacks should be planned for because inevitably, the need to eat a snack will pop up during the course of the day. Planning a snack ahead ensures that an individual doesn't over-indulge and also ensures that healthy foods still enter the body system.

- ***Rule# 4: Avoid second servings***

  To keep extra weight off, Keto practitioners must learn to stick to their diet plan and avoid second servings. Remember weight loss principle #2: moderation.

The Role of Exercise in Keto Diets

Many say that one of the best things about using Keto diets for weight loss is that Keto practitioners are not required to follow a workout plan in order to lose weight. This makes the Keto diet so appealing to many because not everyone likes to workout and others simply don't have the time. The question now is, is this "no exercise" claim true?

It is true. Indeed, a Keto diet is one of the few safe ways that anybody can use to effectively lose weight without the need to exercise. This is because when the body is in a state of Ketosis, fat is used as the main source of energy. This means that even while resting, fat storage in the body is used up, providing a trimmer figure.

The next section is a short explanation concerning why the Keto diet works perfectly without the need to even exercise.

Ketosis Induces Constant Fat Burning

In short, Keto practitioners are not required to add exercise to their daily routine but they can still lose weight at a really good rate. There are two reasons why Keto diets work this way, which is not the same as how low-fat diet works.

First, as mentioned in the first chapter, the core of the Keto diet is Ketosis – that vital body state where fat, derived from all possible sources of food, is crucial in fat burning. It uses fat from food and fat stored in the body to convert to energy. Energy is important because it is what keeps the body going. Exercise, daily tasks, conscious activities; pretty much everything the body does uses up energy. Yes, even sleeping uses up energy as the body needs energy to breathe. With all these activities, the body requires more fat to burn as energy. As a result, there's no need to exercise just to burn fat stored in the body.

Second, the fundamental nature of the Keto diet curbs and suppresses appetite. As a result, Keto practitioners do not notice that their calorie intake is reduced because they are eating less. In short, the calorie use of Keto practitioners exceeds their calorie intake thus, practically eliminating the need to exercise.

However, because of the way the Keto diet works, if Keto practitioners do exercise, it provides them with better results as compared to exercising on a low-fat traditional diet. For example, low-fat high-carb dieters who exercise, need around 20 minutes of cardio workout to reach the fat burning zone. Keto practitioners on the other hand, are always in that zone so their weight loss potential is much higher.

Exercises for Keto practitioners can also help them gain muscles, which are more effective in converting fat into energy. This all means that whenever possible, Keto practitioners should add a little bit of exercise routines to help them achieve better results.

Exercise Tips for Starters

After a bout of Keto-flu, the body will start to adjust and adapt to Ketosis. When this happens, it's advisable to begin to add some exercises to the diet. Start with 30 minutes of easy cardio workouts like swimming or walking at least 3 times a week. As the diet progresses, add some resistance training, which can improve lean muscle gain. Monitor weight changes and when it does improve, increase the workout intensity.

Recap

In summary, here are the things one must do in a Keto diet:

- ### *Create a workable and practical diet plan*

  It's not easy to stick to a Keto diet or to any diet for that matter, without a plan, especially for busy people. With a diet plan however, practitioners can still apply the diet even when they are in school, at work, or anywhere else. Make sure that a diet plan is achievable.

- ### *Reduce carbs and remove totally if possible*

  It's important to follow the general rule of Keto diets. Low carbs and high fats are the driving force for this diet. However, if potential practitioners find it hard to adhere to 20 grams of carbs a day, they can start at their normal levels and gradually reduce to 20 grams. For example, a person can start at 100 grams and gradually reduce 10 grams from it on a daily basis until the recommended 20 grams is achieved. Tip: always check nutrition labels. Many people are surprised to find out that carb-free foods are not what they seem until they check nutrition labels.

- *Always have the essentials on hand*

By the time a Keto diet is embarked upon, staples in a meal plan will include all the foods allowed in the diet such as meat, fatty fish, whole eggs, cheese, oils, nuts, cream and avocados. Making sure there are ample amounts of these foods within reach can help practitioners stick to their diet plans.

- *Complement each meal with vegetables*

Foods high in fat are also high in calories. Because of this, it's important to always add many vegetables low in carbohydrates to any meal.

- *Discover other Keto-friendly foods by doing research*

A Keto meal doesn't always have to be just about meat and vegetables. It can also include pasta, muffins, bread, brownies, ice cream and pudding as long as they are Keto-friendly. These are readily available online or they can be made at home. Search the Internet for alternative recipes.

- **Don't stop searching**

Yes, don't stop searching until that most suitable and lovable version of the diet is found. As mentioned in Chapter 1, there are several versions of Ketogenic diets. Try out each one and stick to which suits one best.

- **Replace what's missing**

There are three ways to replace what's missing: drink lots of water, add salt to meals and take supplements. Ketosis alters the body's water retention and mineral balance. As a result, the body needs more water and salt. Taking Ketone salt supplements is a great way to replace electrolytes lost in the process.

- **Keep a record of everything**

Right from the start, keep track of the body's progress as it undergoes the Keto diet. Take photos, measure parts of the body and monitor changes in weight at least every 3 weeks or on a monthly basis. If there are no improvements, maybe it's time to gradually reduce more carbs, add more fats or add more protein. Another way of knowing if the diet is working is by using Keto sticks. These are strips that test Ketone levels in the blood or urine.

Consistency is important in any diet. It is a major factor that contributes to the success in any diet. If practitioners stick to a Keto diet, they can enjoy both health and weight loss benefits.

Chapter 4
Ketogenic Diet 101:
What Not to Do in a Ketogenic Diet

As with any diet, there are sacrifices to be made. While there are great substitutes to the foods many people love, there's no getting around the fact that there are foods to be avoided in a Keto diet. As the general rule, Keto practitioners should avoid fruits (yes, that's right), starchy foods, wheat (pastas and bread), and pretty much anything that contains refined carbohydrates. Let's look at some foods that Keto practitioners need to give up for good.

Foods to Be Avoided In Keto Diets

In other words, these foods should not be included in Keto diet meal plans.

- *Potatoes*

  The potato is a staple food in many cultures worldwide. It is one of the best food sources available. It can be cooked in many ways and it's even one of the greatest side dishes to ever grace dinner plates. It's also nutritious and delicious to boot. Who doesn't love French fries?!

On the contrary, the potato is murder for those on a Keto diet. Keto practitioners may eat the smallest portions of potato dishes once in a blue moon but such foods have to go away permanently. Here's the reason: potatoes are full of starch. In fact, they are one of the starchiest foods on Earth.

Starch is a carbohydrate and it consists largely of glucose. Remember, a successful Keto diet is one with low carbohydrate and glucose intake. By eating just one large baked potato, the body gets a very high amount of carbohydrates. It doesn't take long for that potato to turn into glucose – sugar, and drive people crazy. People should know that it just doesn't take candy or sugary treats to get sugar levels high.

It's understandable that removing potatoes from meals is hard; it's too much of a staple. However, Keto practitioners will learn in the long run, that potatoes can be substituted with more Keto-friendly foods. For example, instead of pairing a steak with mashed potatoes, do away with green leafy salads.

- *Beans*

  They look harmless but are actually high in carbohydrates. They are actually considered healthy because they also have high amounts of fiber. Their reserve of proteins is also similar to meats. The truth is, they really are great to eat. However, for Keto practitioners, they are not the best of foods. Unlike potatoes though, beans can be eaten in small portions. Still, it depends on the type of dish. Stay away from sweet beans dishes. Bean soups are acceptable.

- *Rice*

  Just like potatoes, rice, (especially the white variety), is full of starch which turns into sugar in the body. As an offender of Keto diets, it is not as bad as potatoes, but it is not to be eaten frequently either. However, brown rice is acceptable in small portions. Unlike white rice, it contains fiber which slows down the process of breaking down carbohydrates and turning it to sugar, producing less strain on the body. It is still high in carbohydrates though, so be careful with this one either way.

- *Sweets*

Do not eat sweets. In other words, do not eat desserts, ice cream, candy and other sugary foods that people use as excuses to cure their sweet cravings. Actually, there's no real reason not to eat sweets in today's world because of all the low-carb substitutes available. Recipes are freely available online and there are a lot of low-carb snacks and foods in grocery stores. However, if planning to eat sweets, (even if they're just substitutes), do it with a plan which is the first step in a Keto diet. Do not give in to cravings. Planning is everything.

- *Fruits*

Like beans, fruits are considered healthy and all-natural. In today's regular diet of white bread, desserts, sodas and pasta however, it becomes too much of a deal. A combination of all the sugars sourced from fruits plus all the sugars from other foods that people eat becomes too much for the body to process properly and will make a person feel awful at the end of the day.

Fruits are better sources of sugar compared to desserts or candy because they have fiber in them. Despite this, Keto practitioners are still discouraged from eating fruits because many of them such as bananas are high in carbohydrates. In short, they have sugar and carbohydrates, a lethal combination for Keto practitioners.

Aside from fruits, stay away from fruit juices. They are the worst kind because fruits are stripped away of their fiber in this state. Eat only those that are allowed in Keto diets as mentioned in Chapter 3. Avoid canned fruits with sugary syrups as well.

- *Bread*

  This part of the diet is quiet surprising. Bread, as long as it's whole-wheat, is allowed. However, it must be loaded with or made into a sandwich with lots of meat, vegetables, and cheese. At the same time, do not eat bread with another major source of carbohydrate, even if it's whole-wheat. For example, do not eat bread and pasta, or bread and French fries, or bread and rice. In general, avoid bagels, doughnuts, rolls, biscuits and other white bread products.

- *Pasta*

Like potatoes, pasta is hard not to include in meals. Everybody loves pasta. Spaghetti anyone? Athletes are even told to load up on pasta for endurance and strength, mainly because pastas are high in carbohydrates. They are mainly made of refined flour. However, they contain very little fiber and nutritional value. They even clog up colons and are mostly just filler in meals. There is absolutely nothing good about pastas. For Keto practitioners, avoid them at all costs.

For those who feel they may not survive without pasta, there are pasta substitutes made of soy. There are also whole-wheat pastas. Unfortunately, they don't taste as good as the real thing. There are also vegetable pastas too, which are good enough.

- *Milk*

Milk is actually high in carbohydrates, but if it is consumed as the main source of carbohydrates in a meal, it wouldn't be that bad. However, many are not easily satisfied with drinking milk alone. They have to pair their milk with something else like cereal for example. Looking closely, an 8-ounce glass of milk contains 12 grams of carbohydrates. A cup of regular cereal contains a whopping 45 grams of carbohydrates. Adding the two, there'll be 57 grams in total and that's more than a day's required supply of carbohydrates in Keto diets.

These foods are especially mentioned because they are major sources of carbohydrates. They are just the tip of the iceberg. There are others that are not allowed in Keto diets such as the following:

Sugary foods	Soda, smoothies (green smoothies are ok), cake, pastries
Highly-processed foods	Cereals, sugar-free foods, low-fat products, frozen cold cuts
Unhealthy fat	Mayonnaise, vegetable oils
Tubers and root vegetables	Parsnips, sweet potatoes, carrots
Beans or legumes	Chickpeas, lentils, kidney beans, peas
Fruits	All fruit, except all kinds of berries
Sauces or condiments	These often contain sugar and unhealthy fat.
Alcohol	All alcoholic drinks

Another important thing to do in a Keto diet is:

Don't Panic!

Aggravation, irritability, poor mental function, dizziness, decreased exercise performance, mental fogginess, headaches, fatigue, digestive discomfort, poor energy, increased hunger and nausea are some of the initial side effects of Keto diets. They are perfectly natural, so don't panic.

The first three days of experiencing these flu-like symptoms – thus called the Keto-flu – are the hardest. To help ease these symptoms, take supplements and add more salt to Keto meals. Take daily doses of:

- *magnesium (300 mg)*

- *potassium (1,000 mg) and*

- *sodium (3,000-4,000 mg)*

As a precaution, consult a doctor first before getting on a Keto diet. On the other hand, why do these adverse effects happen anyway?

The Best Strategy to Manage the Keto Diet's Adverse Effects

As mentioned above, the hard part of adapting to a Keto diet is during its first stages – the time when the initial side effects kick in. There are two reasons why this happen.

First, the body has not yet adapted to its new and main source of energy. Glucose becomes less available and the metabolism of ketones and fat has not yet effectively taken over the body's energy process. Experts suggest that eating a lot of fat is the best strategy for coping with this. Again and again, there is no need to restrict fat intake in this diet, even if practitioners want their body to use up its storage of fat. Go ahead and eat more fat. It is an important source of nutrients and essential fatty acids. Plus, eating more fat with protein helps the body to regulate its insulin response. Remember, a Keto diet is a high-fat diet, not a high-protein diet. There's no need to fear fat. As the body adapts in the first stages of Keto diet, eat plenty of fat to ensure there is enough energy available.

The second reason why adverse effects happen is a result of the temporary rapid water loss and sodium excretion as mentioned in Chapter 3. As a result, both potassium and sodium are lost too quickly if no care is taken to replenish water and sodium. This can lead to headaches, weakness and tiredness. To help prevent these symptoms, make sure to get enough sodium: about 2 teaspoons of table salt or 5 grams of supplements per day.

While magnesium deficiency can cause dizziness and fatigue as well as muscle cramps, a potassium deficiency will cause a person to experience loss of lean body mass. Meat is an abundant source of both magnesium and potassium. However these minerals are easily lost if meat is cooked in water, especially if the meat was boiled. These minerals can end up in the drippings of meat so do not boil meat or cook it in water. Make sure to preserve all the meat's liquids. In addition, severe effects can be cut short by taking magnesium and potassium supplements. At the same time, regular drinking of meat broth is highly recommended.

Finally, at a minimum, symptoms can stay for as little as 4 or 5 days. However, it takes 2 weeks or more to fully adapt to metabolic changes. Keep dietary carbohydrates low. Being in a Keto diet does not mean a person can experiment with carbohydrate tolerance or try out other foods when not sure about their carbohydrate content. The worst scenario is eating some more every few days and then eating less on other days. This can set anybody back. Commit to a low carbohydrate intake, and stick with it. Be consistent until Ketone production is in full force and even when that level is reached, keep it up.

Chapter 5:
A Ketogenic Meal Plan

Here is a week's worth of Keto meals to help beginners kick-start their diet. This 1-week diet plan is made up of simple low-carb meals that anybody can prepare and enjoy. This can also be used as a guide in creating a Keto diet meal plan.

A Sample Keto Meal Plan for Starters

Days	Meals
Day 1	Breakfast: cream cheese pancakes Egg, goat cheese, tomato and basil omelet (optional) Coffee with heavy cream and no-carb sweetener
	Snack: half avocado with lite salt (with potassium) and pepper 1 cup salted chicken broth
	Lunch: chicken salad with feta cheese and olive oil

	Green smoothie with strawberries
	Snack: 2-3 string cheese
	Dinner: green leafy salad with olive oil
	Pork chops with broccoli and parmesan cheese
	(Optional) Dessert: 1 serving of chocolate mousse
Day 2	Breakfast: tomato slices and 3-cheese omelet
	Sausage
	(optional) Coffee with heavy cream and no-carb sweetener
	Snack: a handful of almonds
	Lunch: Shrimp salad with avocado and olive oil
	Green smoothie with blueberries
	Snack: half avocado with lite salt and pepper
	Dinner: steamed salmon with buttered asparagus

	(Optional) Dessert: 1 serving chocolate truffles
Day 3	Breakfast: ham and cheese omelet with onions and peppers
	Cream cheese pancakes
	(optional) Coffee with heavy cream and no-carb sweetener
	Snack: 2 tablespoons peanut butter
	Lunch: bun-less burger with salsa, guacamole, and cheese
	Green smoothie with raspberries
	Snack: a handful of walnuts
	Dinner: beef steak, vegetables and cheese
	(Optional) Dessert: 1 serving low-carb blueberry cheesecake
Day 4	Breakfast: two sausages
	low-carb pancakes
	(optional) Coffee with heavy cream and no-

	carb sweetener
	Snack: a handful of nuts
	Lunch: low-carb bread with lunchmeat, 1 tomato slice and cheese
	Green smoothie with blackberries
	Snack: bowl of cottage cheese with raspberries
	Dinner: salad with roast beef
	Dill pickle
Day 5	Breakfast: tomato slices
	Ham and scrambled eggs
	(optional) Coffee with heavy cream and no-carb sweetener
	Snack: 2-3 crackers with cream cheese
	Lunch: 2-3 fried salmon patties
	Green smoothie with blueberries

	Snack: a handful of nuts
	Dinner: chicken barbeque and salad
	Bowl of strawberries (about 8-10 pieces)
	(Optional) Dessert: low-carb muffins
Day 6	Breakfast: egg omelet with green peppers, onions, cheese and ham
	(optional) Coffee with heavy cream and no-carb sweetener
	Snack: bowl of cottage cheese with blueberries
	Lunch: salad in a low-carb tortilla
	Cottage cheese and 2 fresh peaches
	Snack: 2-3 slices of cheddar cheese
	Dinner: beef jerky and salad
	Celery with cream cheese
	Tomato slices
	(Optional) Dessert: low-carb muffins

Day 7	Breakfast: low-carb bread with slices of cheese and chicken breast
	(optional) Coffee with heavy cream and no-carb sweetener
	Snack: a handful of almonds
	Lunch: meat loaf with salad
	Snack: crackers with cheese
	Dinner: fried fish fillet and 1/2 cup of brown rice
	Green beans
	(Optional) Dessert: 1 serving of low-carb strawberry cream pie

Aside from the foods mentioned in this diet plan, here are some more foods that can be added in a Keto diet plan:

Food Group	Kinds
Vegetables	Swiss chard, cabbage, zucchini, celery, mushrooms, green beans, asparagus, Brussels sprouts, kale, spinach, bell peppers, cucumber, eggplant, cauliflower
Meats	lamb, turkey, veal, venison, bison
Fish and seafood	sardines, trout, shellfish, catfish cod, halibut, tuna, lobster, herring, haddock
Fruits and berries	mulberries, oranges, kiwi, lemons, apricots, grapefruit
Nuts and seeds	chia seeds, pumpkin seeds, flaxseeds, pistachios, cashews, macadamia nuts,

	hazelnuts, sunflower seeds
Dairy foods	Greek yoghurt, full-fat yoghurt
Fats and oils	coconut oil, tallow, lard, avocado oil
Beverages	tea, sugar-free carbonated drinks, green smoothies
Chocolate	Dark chocolate
Condiments, herbs, and spices	oregano, mustard, cinnamon, ginger, garlic

Meanwhile, here are some Keto-friendly snack ideas. Snack on these treats when feeling hungry in between meals.

1. Remember those leftover foods from yesterday's meals? They are perfect snack treats for Keto practitioners. Nibble on those few slices of chicken breast, or barbecued pork chops.

2. Vegetable sticks dipped in salsa, guacamole, peanut butter, or cream cheese are all delicious and nutritious. Cucumbers, celery, or some zucchini dipped in guacamole are heavenly.

3. A bowl of Keto-friendly fruits with the occasional heavy cream is also perfect.

4. A combination of cheese and Keto-friendly fruits.

5. Hard-boiled eggs.

6. A few strips of beef jerky.

7. Keto-friendly fruits with Greek or full-fat yoghurt are really good.

This diet plan is pretty basic, but there are many options available out there. Just remember the diet restrictions discussed in the previous chapter and the foods allowed in Chapter 3.

Also, this diet plan is not hard to modify. Anyone can improve this plan to suit their personal preferences. Always try to rotate meats and vegetables to create delicious combinations.

Chapter 6:
Does Anyone Have a Question?

Drawing on the materials that were discussed in the previous chapters, here are some important and anticipated questions that readers might ask, with corresponding answers.

- ***Is this diet safe in general?***

  This is a fair question. It wouldn't help if individuals practiced Keto diets but eventually began to suffer. In relation to this question, the two biggest concerns individuals face in Keto diets are:

  1. Will I suffer nutritionally?

  2. Will it raise my cholesterol levels, leading to a heart attack?

  These questions are perfectly understandable considering the high-fat requirement of Keto diets. However, these questions have been thoroughly answered by numerous studies done over the last decade. Many studies reveal that a low-carb, high-fat diet does not raise cholesterol levels in the body. In fact, the total cholesterol in the body decreases while it undergoes a Keto diet. Medical experts pushing for low-fat diets are bewildered that people would want to try this diet and keep insisting that Keto diets are crazy. To their surprise, people who eat low-carb meals show improvements in all their major health indicators.

In a Keto diet, practitioners are expected to eat more protein and are therefore, expected to take more cholesterol in. However, this does not mean that practitioners will be loading their bodies with cholesterol. They can eat all the meat and salads they want for the rest of their lives but still keep their triglycerides low. What raises cholesterol is the pairing of fatty foods with carbohydrates and that's when people become candidates for heart attacks.

- *Does this mean I can eat all the red meat I want?*

Studies show that red meat, when eaten in Keto diets, is actually not the problem that low-fat, high-carbs experts say they are. As long as individuals keep their carb intake at low levels, they can enjoy all the hamburgers, meat loaves, bacon, steaks and barbeques they want. Having said that, moderation is a principle (Weight

Loss Principle#2) that Keto dieters should always practice. At the same time, don't just eat only red meat. Eat fish, chicken, turkey and other meats as well, as long as they're Keto-friendly. The reasonable approach here is to avoid extremes. Don't overload on red meat but don't be afraid of it either. Remember that the real danger is when a person eats lots of red meat and then eats lots of carbs too.

- **I have diabetes, is this diet good for me?**

Of course! The Ketogenic has been found to be beneficial most especially for people with metabolism disorders.

- **My friend has no diabetes, is this diet also good for her?**

There is no suitable diet for everyone because all humans differ in personal preferences, tastes, lifestyles, body types, genes and metabolism. People who don't like foods high in fats but want to keep carbs in their diet may find it hard to stick to a Keto diet. A standard low-carb diet or carb-cycling is most suitable for them. The Standard Keto version is also not suitable for vegans or vegetarians due to its high-fat requirement. The Standard Keto diet is also not suitable for athletes or for those who wish to gain muscles. The Cyclical or Targeted Keto versions are more suitable for them.

- **Does this mean I can lose muscle or I can't build muscles?**

  Actually, there's a chance individuals can lose muscle in any diet not just in Keto diets. However, for individuals who are in Keto diets and include weight-lifting in their workout regimen, high Ketone levels and high protein intake can minimize muscle loss.

  Individuals can also build muscles with Keto diets, though the muscle gain is not as effective when compared to other diets. Individuals who wish to stick with Keto diets but also want to build muscles can use the Targeted of Cyclical versions of Keto diets.

- **I want to lose weight quickly, is a Keto diet good for me?**

  Yes. Not only can the Keto diet help people lose fat quickly, it can also help people improve their health. However, it requires discipline and a strict diet plan-compliance.

- *I have started the diet, and now I'm not feeling energized. Is this normal?*

Yes, it's pretty normal. As mentioned in Chapter 4, practitioners will experience Keto-flu at the start of the diet. Hang in there! It'll be worth it in the end. Just wait for it and take supplements.

- *Is it okay to stop eating carbs? Where can I get my energy source now?*

First of all, a Keto diet is not a no-carb diet. Let's clear that out. It's a low-carb diet. Second, even though it's true that carbohydrates are a major source of energy, a little-known fact is that the energy they provide is temporary. They can boost energy levels and blood sugar levels but they can also drop blood sugar levels at an alarming rate, which leaves the body weak and hungry. It's a vicious cycle.

A healthier option is to eat vegetables and some fruits, which surprisingly, have carbohydrates in them. Low-carb foods are also available in grocery stores and can be ordered online.

- **Will I ever get the chance to eat actual carbs again?**

Yes, of course. At the start of Keto diets, major sources of carbohydrates must be temporarily eliminated. After the body adapts to the diet well enough, which takes about 2-3 months, individuals can eat actual carbs again, though occasionally only. The Keto diet is not a one-time diet method; it's a lifestyle. For example, if practitioners eat pasta for lunch today, it must be followed by a low-carb or no-carb meal for dinner.

- **Where can I get low-carb substitutes or recipes?**

Today, majority of low-carb foods can be bought from health-food stores and on the Internet. However, some grocery stores have specialty foods section which offer low-carb alternatives.

- **Do I really have to give up eating fruits?**

Not at all. However, practitioners are advised to be wise and careful in choosing fruits. Low-carb fruits should be emphasized in Keto diets. Berries and melons are excellent choices as well as small tangerines are great because of their low carbohydrate content. They are a good source of vitamin C too. Fruit juices are a no-no, however. Stripped of their fiber, they easily become sugar in the body. Some fruits meanwhile, are quite high in carbohydrates such as large oranges, apples and bananas. They can be eaten but sparingly. It is recommended to eat them in halves only.

There are Keto-friendly fruits that practitioners can eat. Please refer to Chapter 3 for a list of foods to eat for Keto dieters.

- **Speaking of fruits, my urine smells fruity. Is this normal?**

Yes, it is normal to have fruity-smelling urine while on Keto diets. There's no need to be alarmed. This happens because Ketosis expels by-products and these cause the fruity scent.

- **My breath smells too, though not fruity. Is this normal, too?**

This is a common side effect of increased fat intake. Repel the bad smell by chewing sugar-free gum or drinking naturally-flavored water.

- *I experience digestion problems while on a Keto diet. Is this normal?*

  Not all Keto practitioners experience this phase but it's normal. It's a known side effect but it typically passes after 3 weeks to 1 month. If it persists, take magnesium supplements to ease constipation and eat more vegetables or high-fiber foods.

The author hopes that this e-book has answered all questions about Keto diets concisely. Now, before closing this chapter and the e-book finally, let's do a recap of how to effectively lose weight using the Ketogenic Diet.

Note: Choosing a suitable version of Keto diet should've been the first step. However, SKD, or the standard Keto diet is the subject of this book, so we're using it as the basis for this summary.

- *Step 1*

  Create a list of foods that are allowed and not allowed in Keto diets. This will be the basis for creating diet plans.

- ***Step 2***

  Create a diet plan based on the list of foods mentioned above. Make sure to include snacks in the plan.

- ***Step 3***

  Minimize carbohydrate intake, eat enough proteins and add more fats in the diet plan. Remember, the general rule is: 5% carbs (20-30 grams) + 70% fats + 25% protein. Start with this and adjust accordingly as the diet progress.

- ***Step 4***

  Keep track of all the changes that happen, from the start point to current status. Use Keto sticks to determine if Ketosis is activated already. Typically, this can happen after 2 weeks. For shorter periods, eat less and less carbs, about 15 grams only.

- ***Step 5***

  The body will undergo Keto-flu as soon as it enters the Ketosis state. Remember, don't panic. It's all part of the diet and in the end, it's all worth it. Hang in there!

- ***Step 6***

  Add more water and salt to the diet plan. As soon as the body enters Ketosis, it will lose more water and electrolytes. Replenish them religiously. Otherwise, the body will experience headaches, panic attacks, palpitations and nausea.

- ***Step 7***

  After adapting to the changes that Ketosis brings, include exercises in the diet. A regimen can be simple aerobic exercises, jogging or walking. Do not exercise on an empty stomach, though.

- ***Step 8***

  Stay on track. Keep the weight off by using the Keto diet as a lifestyle. It not only benefits weight management, it also offers numerous other health benefits.

Overall, eating low amount of carbs, moderate protein and a high amount of fat can have an enormous impact in anybody's health. It lowers blood sugar, body weight and cholesterol. It even raises energy and mood levels.

Conclusion

I hope this book was able to help you to understand more about the benefits of the Ketogenic Diet and its contribution to weight loss efforts.

The next step is to start a diet and exercise plan, stick with it and when you reach a goal, reward yourself.

If you enjoyed this book, then I'd like to ask you for a favor, would you be kind enough to leave a review for this book on Amazon? It'd be greatly appreciated!

Thank you again for purchasing this book and Good luck!

Made in the USA
San Bernardino, CA
28 October 2016